MORINGA
THE MIRACLE TREE

Nature's Most Powerful
Super Food Revealed

*Natures All In One Plant For
Natural Remedies, Natural
Health and Natural Anti-Aging*

JOY LOUIS

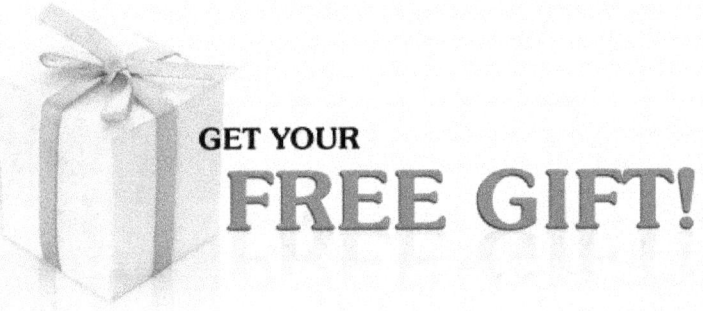

GET YOUR
FREE GIFT!

WAIT! BEFORE YOU CONTINUE –
DO YOU LIKE FREE BOOKS?

My **FREE Gift** to You!! As a way to say **Thank You** for downloading my book, I'd like to offer you more **FREE BOOKS**! Each time we release a NEW book, we offer it first to a small number of people as a test–drive. Because of your commitment here in downloading my book, I'd love for you to be a part of this group. You can join easily here→ **http://goo.gl/4lB2sj**

Do You Enjoy **FREE BOOKS**? Do you like books that are Life Changing, Inspirational, Motivational and Informative? We **LOVE** sharing **FREE BOOKS** with people like you. It's easy to join just by clicking here→ **http://goo.gl/4lB2sj**

FROM AUTHOR JOY LOUIS:

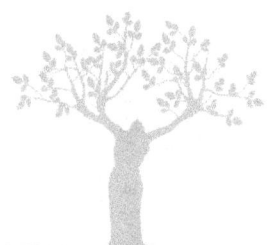

I'm so very excited and honored that you've picked up this book and want to learn more about essential oils!

Before you read on and really dive into the book let me introduce myself...

My name is Joy, and I'm an all Natural-Organic-Homemade "Everything" Person. In other words: I have a natural solution for pretty much everything in my life!

My "all natural" way of living started a few years back when I was sick and tired of being sick, FAT and tired. I was eating pretty healthy (or so I thought): I ate peanut butter jelly sandwiches for lunch every day, snacked on cereal protein bars in between meals (these are healthy, right?) and drank Diet Coke (because isn't Diet Coke better than sugar? No calories versus a mother lode of sugar that would go straight to my butt. I'll take the "no sugar" please and thank you). However, despite living my so-called "healthy" lifestyle, I kept gaining weight, and lost all energy and motivation to do anything; I even started to dread taking my dearest Pretzel (my sweet dog of 7 years) out for her daily walk around the neighborhood!

That's when I knew I'd had enough. I decided to start searching for a better way; a way that has now proven to give me more energy than I ever imagined possible and also helped me lose 45 pounds of stubborn body fat in the process. I made a drastic change, 180-degree turn in all my habits.

So here it is. My so called "secret, hidden formula" I used to get to where I am today is: I went ALL NATURAL. Not a very sexy answer, is it? Well I have to tell you, a lot of times we complicate things way too much when looking for an answer. More often than not the solution to our problems is very simple. However... simple doesn't mean it's easy - far from it!

As for me, I don't know how I gathered the willpower to do this, but somehow I managed to throw out all of my garbage foods (i.e cereal bars, cookies, chips and so on) and replaced them with organic, GMO-free vegetables, fruits and lean meats all within **one** day. I completely went cold turkey: I stopped using all of the popular soaps and lotions out there that are FILLED with toxins, and instead I made my own, or found other safe brands and options. A short time after my big lifestyle change I learned about essential oils, and soon they became a necessity in my every day life. They are such an important part of my life and have helped me so much that I have now written a book about them. The world needs to know about these oils, their healing properties and the overall well-being of the people who use them!

As for myself, I use them in almost everything. They're my go-to problem solver, my all-natural medicine cabinet. No more artificial pain killers or medicine with a hundred possible side effects. Essential oils keep my food cravings in check, clear out my sinuses when feel a cold coming on, straighten out the wrinkles and lines coming on in my face, and uplifts my mood the days I feel anxious. For the first time in my life, I can finally say I feel 100% present and alive! I have started to love my body and I have found a true passion in helping others, hence why I decided to write this book. I truly hope you find this book helpful, and please let me know if you have any questions about any of the content.

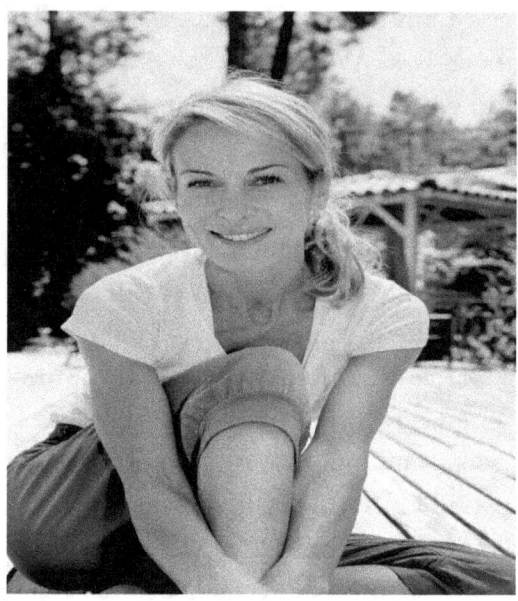

With much love,

Joy Louis

Connect with Joy here:

https://www.facebook.com/JoyLouisBooks

Find more of Joy's books here:

http://www.amazon.com/Joy-Louis/e/B00UMOZJE6

TABLE OF CONTENTS

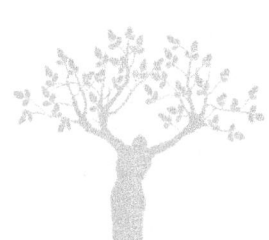

INTRODUCTION

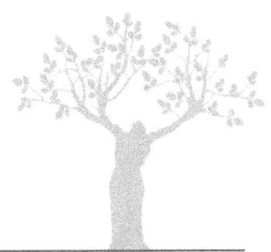

I want to thank you and congratulate you for downloading the book, *"**Moringa Oleifera**: Nature's most Powerful Super Food"*.

Moringa Oleifera is a relatively natural concept in the western world, only rediscovered in the last few decades. Since then, multiple uses of this 'miracle tree' has been found, benefits that stretch from nutrition to health, beauty to hygiene, detoxification to weight loss, and many more. Research is still being done on many more ways that the various parts of this plant can help human kind, and there is more knowledge to come our way.

This book - *Moringa Oleifera: Nature's most Powerful Super Food* - is a complete guide to all things Moringa. It contains everything that you will need to know about Moringa Oleifera, about how and where it grows, how it can help in our nutrition and health, how we can cook it, how we can use it as first aid in our everyday household ailments and troubles, and how you can make beauty and health products with it.

But above all, this book contains an in-depth knowledge of all the nutritional, culinary, health and medicinal properties of the Moringa Oleifera plant.

Thanks again for downloading this book, I hope you enjoy it!

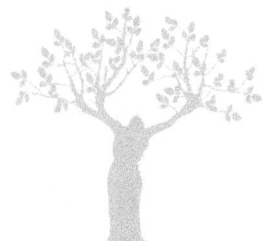

Chapter 1

ALL ABOUT MORINGA OLEIFERA

While we go on with our busy and hectic life, making ourselves sick with worrying about our careers, our lives, our relationships and our future, we are also harming ourselves greatly by another folly - eating the way we eat.

The way the modern population gouges on processed and packaged food, carbohydrates and unhealthy fats effect greatly on our physique - greatly and negatively. Not only does what we eat cause obesity and heart problems, but also problems with our blood pressure, cholesterol, nutrition deficiency, and even some mental and emotional distress.

However, thanks to nature that there is always a treasure of super food available to mankind which the human body actually needs and which can help us maintain our health and sanity. Not only that, these super foods are so incredible in their nutritional values and properties, that they have the power to heal, and to save us from the physical pit that we have put ourselves.

Moringa Oleifera is one such gift of nature to humankind - a super food that almost has all the answers.

If this is the first time that you are hearing of Moringa Oleifera, it is extremely normal. This is not a food that is as common as carrots or oatmeal, especially not in the western world, but it is extremely beneficial to the human body and to our health.

This book can be considered as the complete guide to Moringa Oleifera - everything that you would need to know about this super food found in nature, including its various uses, its properties, its health benefits and especially, the different ways to eat it.

ALL ABOUT MORINGA OLEIFERA

Surprisingly, Moringa Oleifera is not a fruit; neither is it a vegetable nor a grain. This super food available in nature is actually a plant, and it is possible to use every part of this plant – from its leaves to its root and flowers.

Almost no other food available in nature is so full of nutrition and benefits as the Moringa Oleifera. While fruits like oranges and lemons are abundant in calcium and vegetables like spinach is known for it's iron contents, Moringa, surprisingly, doesn't fall in just any one category of nutrition. Astoundingly, this food contains a high amount of almost every type of nutrition that is available and needed in human beings. That is why it is sometimes called 'Nature's most Important Super Food'.

Let's know some more about this super food before learn of its benefits and uses.

ORIGIN AND HISTORY

Moringa Oleifera is a native of the Himalayas in Northern India, and later spread towards the other tropical and sub-tropical regions of the subcontinent, including China, the Philippines and the other nearby countries of Asia.

The word 'Moringa' is derived from the Tamil word *'Murungai'*. It is more commonly known as the *'Horse-Radish Tree'* in the western world because of the condiment that is prepared from its roots; sometimes it is also known as the *'Drumstick tree'* because of the shape of the pods.

Some other names of this plant are the *'Ben Oil Tree'*, *'Kelor'* and *'Malunggay'*.

In ancient times, Moringa was cultivated as far as Egypt and the Mesopotamian areas, where references to this tree have been made in 2000 BC, calling it 'the miracle tree'.

Moringa Oleifera was a prized and expensive plant in ancient Rome and Greece.

AVAILABILITY AND CULTIVATION

India is the largest producer of Moringa in the world, especially the southern regions of Andra Pradesh, Karnataka and Tamil Nadu.

The farmers of Thailand, Haiti, Taiwan and Philippines grow Morinaga to be sold in the local markets for various uses. In the recent years, the production of this plant has reached Central America, the Caribbean Islands, some countries of North and South America and Africa as well as Oceania.

Despite having the perfect climate and soil to produce this plant in many regions of the world, not many countries are aware of the wonderful benefits of this plant.

Moringa Oleifera requires tropical, subtropical and semiarid areas to be cultivated, with land that is slightly acidic, loamy and sandy. It prefers a hot and sunny weather, and can be irrigated with rainwater.

DESCRIPTION

As we mentioned before, Moringa Oleifera is actually a plant and it is possible to use every part of this plant to our advantage. A fully grown plant can reach up to 35-40 feet in height with a diameter of 1.5 feet.

The flowers from this plant are fragrant and can bloom up to 0.5 inches in length.

Multiple fruits, or the Moringa pods, hang from the plant and are 25-40 cm in length, resembling a three-sided capsule. The fruits/pods resemble long and thin beans, or pea pods. They are green and soft when young but gradually turn hard and brown.

Each pod holds multiple dark brown seeds, each one 1 cm in diameter, ranging from 5 to 20 seeds, depending on the size of the pod. Each of the seeds has three wing-like structures which are papery and white. The seeds are used for further cultivation and breeding.

BREEDING AND YIELD

Moringa can be breed and planted through direct seeding or cuttings; it is very easy to be transferred or germinated to a new region with favorable conditions. In its native land India, Moringa

Oleifera grows wild and in abundance. In other countries, the production is comparatively smaller but shows promise.

Moringa Oleifera is cultivated for its leaves, roots, pods and kernels as well as its flowers and fruits. The first harvest can take 6-8 months after the first planting, except for the fruits which usually takes one year to appear.

For all its nutritional values and many benefits and uses, Moringa Oleifera has earned the title of 'Nature's most Powerful Super food'. Let's find out a few uses of this plant in our daily lives.

Chapter 2

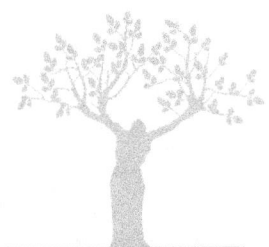

USES OF MORINGA OLEIFERA

Though this plant is not very well known in the western world, its various parts can be used in almost all aspects of our lives. This plant has earned the title of 'Nature's most powerful super food' for one reason, and that is its positive role and importance in the betterment of our life in every way possible.

Since Moringa Oleifera is a plant and most commonly, an edible plant, it's main uses are in the kitchen as a culinary assistant. Not so much in the western countries, but in the Asian subcontinent and many African countries, Moringa is considered a delicacy and an everyday cuisine.

Besides being an appetizing dish, Moringa is also used for detoxification of the body and as an ingredient to encourage weight loss.

Also, Moringa is used for various other health and beauty purposes. We will discuss each aspect of its usefulness in details in this chapter.

I. MORINGA: A CULINARY MARVEL

Moringa is considered a delicacy in the Indian Subcontinent and in many countries of Asia and Africa and is a everyday part of the meal plans of the local people, especially in the rural areas where Moringa is found and grown in abundance.

The most common parts of the Moringa plant that is eaten as food are the leaves, the pods (the fruits) and the seeds. Some people also eat the flowers which are an important part of the cuisine in some Asian countries.

The roots are also used in cooking; however, they are concentrated in flavors and elements and should not be taken in a large amount directly.

MORINGA PODS

The pods of the Moringa tree - when immature and green - are used as a vegetable to cook into a spicy curry and eaten during any meal. Green Moringa pods are cooked into soup, which preserves all its nutrients in the gravy.

In some areas, the immature Moringa is boiled to soften them up, and consumed directly as a vegetable. However, boiling the Moringa pods looses almost all its nutrients, especially if the excess water is thrown away.

In the Asian countries, Moringa pods are cooked as curry with other vegetables, separately or with fish, and eaten with rice or *chapati* (bread), especially in the Indian subcontinent.

The soft and flavorful inner-flesh of the green pods is sometimes separated from the pods to be added to soups, *dal* (lentil), *sambar* (chowder) or other similar curries. This increases the flavor of the dishes and adds extra nutrition to them. These dishes are more popular in India, Bangladesh and Pakistan.

The young and soft seeds are also used to add to the flavor in soups and curries.

MORINGA FLOWERS

The flowers taste similar to mushrooms when cooked as curry. They are also dipped in spiced *besan* (gram flour) and deep-fried in oil to be served as snacks. The flowers can be used in the preparation of lasagna, pancakes, omelets, casseroles, pizza or quiche.

Moringa flowers can also be brewed briefly in tea that can act as a mild laxative. They can also be chopped to be made into a salad with adequate seasonings.

MORINGA LEAVES

Moringa leaves can be eaten raw, dried, cooked or powdered.

The young leaves can be fried to be eaten, or chopped finely to be cooked with fish and soup. Several dishes cooked and loved in Cambodia uses the leaves in their special vegetable and fish soup. The immature leaves are also chopped to be used as garnish in salads and vegetables, like coriander leaves.

The most valuable way to eat the Moringa leaves is by drying them in the sun and crushing them into powder. This powder is extremely versatile and can be consumed in any way and added to anything. It can be eaten directly, mixed with a glass of water or any other drink. This powdered Moringa leaf can also be added to any dish while cooking to ensure extra flavor and nutrition. However, the powder should be added at the end of the cooking so that the nutrition doesn't diminish due to the excess heat.

7 pounds of fully-grown or fresh Moringa leaves, after drying, makes around 1 pound of powder that will keep a family nutritionally sustained for a long time. An adult needs to consume not more than 2 to 3 teaspoon of Moringa powder every day; slightly more than that is also acceptable. However, it is advisable that a person takes in small doses at the beginning, and slowly increases its intake amount.

Moringa leaves can also be used to make juice, baked with other food, added to healthy shakes or in baby food.

MORINGA SEEDS

The seeds of the Moringa tree are one of the most important parts of the tree, especially since it is the main source of breeding. However, Moringa seeds are also valued for their nutritional properties.

Green and immature Moringa seeds that are found inside the pods can be eaten directly, or friend and popped in olive oil, like popcorn. Locals from the countries that grow Moringa regularly eat around 4/5 Moringa seeds everyday to keep up with their daily nutritional needs. Although, more than that everyday can lead to nausea and sleeplessness, since Moringa seeds have some special attributes that are intense and powerful.

Moringa seeds can be added to soups, sauces, curries and stews to be cooked. They can also be dried and added to muffin or bread mixes for baking. Young seeds, boiled in water, or cooked in butter and salted, can also be served as a snack, in small doses.

The most important yield from the seeds of the Moringa tree is the oil that is obtained by pressing them. The oil is odorless and clear, contains important nutrition and elements, and used in many culinary purposes, such as in sauces, as base for mayonnaise, as cooking oil, for garlic bed, and to make popcorn and pasta.

As we can see from this chapter, the Moringa plant can be used in almost all aspects of cooking and consumption. We have included a few interesting and extremely delicious recipes that require the different parts of the Moringa plant at the end of this book that you can try at home.

MORINGA ROOTS

Of all the parts of the Moringa plant, the roots are the only parts which are not supposed to be directly eaten as they contain all of the elements of the entire plant in a concentrated form and a severe proportion. Consuming the roots directly will actually harm the body, especially if eaten in a large amount or for a long time. The roots will be especially harmful during pregnancy or lactation.

The roots of the Moringa are shredded down into little pieces or crushed into powder and used in small doses as a condiment in cooking. Just the minimum amount of Moringa roots while cooking - since it has a strong taste that resembles horseradish - is enough for the nutritional needs of the entire family.

II. MORINGA: HEALTH BENEFITS

In most countries of the world, Moringa Oleifera is consumed as a source of essential nutrition. However, there are also some other uses of this *miracle tree* that helps develop and maintain our health and overall wellbeing.

Different parts of the Moringa plant has been used as home remedies and medicine for simple and daily ailments for a long time. These health benefits of the Moringa tree are well-known in many urban and rural localities in many countries of the world, and have been handed down from generation to generation.

MORINGA FLOWERS

Juice made from the flowers of the Moringa tree is drank in many countries around the world as it is known to increase the flow of breast milk in lactating mothers. It is especially practiced in underdeveloped and developing countries where both the mothers and infants suffer from malnourishment and do not have enough to eat. Moringa flower juice is known to both increase the quality and the quantity of breast milk in mothers.

Moringa flower, after being boiled in water for only 5 minutes, is drunk as tea as a remedy for severe cold in the rural areas of Haiti. It can be boiled with just water, or with tea leaves to give it an extra flavor.

Both Moringa flower juice and tea are taken by people, especially women, who are suffering from UTI, or Urinary Tract

Infection, as the elements in this flower encourages frequent urination.

MORINGA LEAVES

Green and young Moringa leaves are crushed by hand and the pulp is applied on the forehead and temples to get relief from severe headaches and migraine pains in many rural areas. It is the cooling effect of the plants that help in relieving from headache pains.

Tea made with Moringa leaves is drunk by patients suffering from gastric ulcer as well as diarrhea. In Malawi, Africa the leaves of the Moringa tree are dried and eaten to cure severe diarrhea.

Moringa leaves are significantly anti-bacterial and anti-inflammatory, and are therefore used as first aid in cases of minor cuts and bruises. Poultices made of Moringa leaves are effective on minor wounds to stop bleeding. They are also used to treat insect bites and accident wounds.

Juice made from the fresh leaves is known to treat and reduce anxiety in any adverse situation, or in a nervous person.

MORINGA PODS (FRUITS)

In many developing countries, the pods or the fruits of the Moringa plant is eaten to fight the level of malnutrition after a severe case of diarrhea. Also, raw Moringa fruits are eaten to ease joint pain.

MORINGA SEED AND SEED OIL

Roasted Moringa seeds are eaten as a snack to encourage frequent and painless urination, especially by people who suffer from Urinary Tract Infection. The oil extracted from the seeds is also used as a relaxant for epileptic patients.

In many localities of Oman, Moringa seed oil is consumed to treat an upset stomach.

Moringa oil is also used to relax a hysteric person.

MORINGA ROOTS, GUM AND BARK

In villages of India and Senegal, the roots of the Moringa tree is pounded, mixed with pure salt and used as poultice for relief in arthritis pain and rheumatism. The same poultice is also used for kidney pains.

The bark helps to increase appetite and also works as a digestive.

III. MORINGA: BEAUTY SECRETS

Over many years, in many countries of Asia and Africa, Moringa Oleifera has been used in enhancing beauty and preserving health. It is especially the seeds and the oil from the seeds of the Moringa plant that are used in many aspects of health and beauty.

MORINGA SEEDS AND SEED OIL

The seeds that are found inside the pods, i.e. the fruits, of the Moringa tree are pressed to obtain oil which is known as *'Behen Oil'* or *'Ben Oil'*. This is because this oil is rich in *Behenic Acid*, which is a fatty kind of acid.

The Moringa Seed Oil is pale-yellow in color and has a shelf age of more than 5 years. The oil doesn't dry off due to the anti-oxidants present in it that act as natural preservatives. It is rich in fatty acid, Vitamin A, Vitamin C, and various kinds of other essential acids.

This oil is used in cooking purposes in some localities, but its main contribution is in the field of health and beauty. Moringa seed oil is known to show positive effects in the beautification of skin, hair and other parts of the body.

Moringa Oil is known to be:

- Anti aging,

- Anti bacterial,

- Anti inflammatory and

- Anti septic.

From ancient times, Moringa oil has been used as numerous cosmetics to moisture, cleanse, condition and maintain the human body.

For its miraculous anti-aging properties, Moringa oil is used in numerous cosmetic cosmetics in creams, lotions, ointments and oils. It is known to be extremely effective in:

- Reducing visible wrinkle lines,

- Revitalizing dull and tired skin,

- Reversing the aging process,

- Stabilizing Collagen in the skin with the help of the Vitamin C present in the oil,

- Preventing the sagging of the skin due to age,

- Rejuvenate the skin,

- Reducing the fine lines around the face and neck,

- Repairing damaged skin cells,

- Fighting damage of skin tissue that lead to wrinkles,

- Delay damage of skin cells and tissue, and

- Supplying the needed antioxidant and nutrient needed in the skin.

All of which leads to a younger looking face and skin that defies age and time.

Moringa Oil has certain healing effects which help to reduce and cure blemishes, blackheads and pimples. It is used in treating teenage and adult acne as a cleanser, and helps to fight infection and scarring because of its antiseptic properties.

Moringa seed Oil is also used as a carrier oil - a base oil that can be mixed with other essential oils, such as argon, jojoba, coconut and sesame, to be used to make massage oils, natural perfumes and aromatherapy oils. Moringa oil - being light, odorless and yet emollient - is perfect as the base for all these essential oils to be mixed with and used.

This oil is also known for its use on dry skin, as it helps to soften the skin and maintain moisture in the skin.

It is also good for treating skin conditions such as eczema, psoriasis and dermatitis due to its moisturizing nature.

A unique feature of Moringa oil is the ease with which it is absorbed into the skin, leaving it radiant and improved. For this reason, this oil is one of the main ingredients in the preparation of various nature-based creams, lotions, ointments, soaps and body wash, body oils, face creams and lip balms.

Moringa oil, mixed with other carrier oil, is used in hair care to strengthen hair. This oil can be massaged into the scalp to be quickly absorbed into the scalp to release the essential vitamins and minerals that is present in abundance in the oil. It is also useful to moisturize and treat dry and flaky scalp that itches.

Moringa oil is also affective in fighting dandruff by moisturizing the scalp and making the hair roots stronger. It is also good for treating split ends and hair fall. Massaging this oil on damp hair has shown good results for a number of users of Moringa Seed Oil.

Moringa oil is sometimes used in lip balms or applied directly to the lips, in small amounts and mixed with other carrier oils, to treat chapped and dry lips.

Some other beauty benefits of Moringa Oil include:

- Massaging Moringa oil to nails to strengthen cuticles and nail beds.

- Mixing Moringa oil with other carrier oils, i.e. coconut or jojoba oil, to use as toner on the skin.

- Mixing Moringa oil to coconut oil and tea-tree oil to use as natural makeup remover.

- Mixing with natural brown sugar to be used as homemade scrub to exfoliate facial skin and the skin of elbows, knees, heels and back.

- Massaging into acne affected skin to remove pigmentation and scarring.

- Using as facial cleanser to gently clean dirt, oil and pollution from skin pores, leaving them open and manageable.

MORINGA LEAVES

Moringa leaves contain impressive amounts of sulphur which keeps the skin soft and flexible. These leaves, being made into a paste - if applied to the skin as face mask - enhance the brightness of the skin and beautify the tone of the face.

The leaves of the Moringa tree contains as many as 30 types of antioxidants which, by massaging, is delivered into the skin cells and contributes to a healthy, glowing skin.

MORINGA FLOWERS

Moringa flowers are also used to make perfumes and hair oils. It is also used as fragrance for cosmetics and in aromatherapy.

It is the unique combination of nutrition, vitamins and minerals present in the Moringa tree that makes it invaluable to almost all aspects of our lives, from its presence in the kitchen to our health and beauty essentials.

IV. MORINGA: A WEIGHT LOSS MIRACLE

Moringa is relatively a new find in modern science and in the western world, but its uses had been varied and manifold in the Eastern, Asian and African countries of the world. One of its important contributions is to enhance the metabolism system of the human body and aid in significant weight loss.

Weight loss - weight loss in an effective, scientific and healthy way, to be specific - has always been a major concern of millions of people all around the world. Fad diets come and go every month, and every week. Some work on specific people, while others have no effect on our weight and more negative effects on our health.

Moringa Oleifera has recently joined the sparse list of nutritional foods that can guarantee healthy and effective weight loss and have gained worldwide acclamation in this regard. It is said to be one of the most effective, as well as one of the most healthiest way to steadily lose unwanted and excessive weight and maintain a healthy physique known to mankind.

However, no parts of the Moringa Oleifera plant claims to be a magic portion which will drastically help you lose all your excessive weight in a few days. No scientist, nutritionist or companies that produce and market Moringa would be able to claim an effect as radical or as attractive as that. Moreover, scientifically, it is extremely harmful for the body to lose a huge amount of weight in a short time, and Moringa does not support that.

But yes! Moringa Oleifera plant can assist a person in losing or shedding all their extra weight. How long would that take?

That actually depends on that specific person's diet, lifestyle, exercise routine and willingness to sacrifice unhealthy food and lose weight.

HOW CAN MORINGA HELP IN LOSING WEIGHT?

All the parts of the Moringa plant, in small doses or big, are nutritious and can be consumed by an adult. The leaves, roots, pods, seeds and the seed oil - every element of the plant is filled with necessary vitamins, minerals, protein and other essential nutrition that is enough to fulfill a huge portion of a person's daily nutritional value.

Does that mean that in order to lose weight, all we need to eat is Moringa all day, every day, until we reach our desired weight goal? No, not necessary. A normal serving of Moringa Oleifera, or substituting it with any other carbohydrate- or protein-based food will do. You could also add some other Moringa oriented food in your diet, such as Moringa tea instead of coffee or tea, Moringa seeds for snacks and Moringa leaves for your vegetable needs.

The healthiest parts of the Moringa Oleifera plants are their leaves when they are green and new. Eating these leaves as a type of vegetable helps lose weight in a number of ways, as described in details below:

- The leaves of the Moringa plant are one of the most important sources of leafy green vegetable that is available in nature today. As we know, green and leafy vegetables are the ultimate source of minerals, proteins and calcium that the body needs and that we consume from other more fattening food items, such as full-fat milk, legumes and meat.

If we include a lot of the green Moringa leaves in our meals every day, we would be taking in all the necessary nutrition that we need for sustaining ourselves, but without the extra fat or carbohydrates that come with other food items.

- Moringa leaves contained a large amount of Vitamin B - a nutrient that helps digestion. This helps in digesting the food you eat everyday quicker so that it can pass on smoothly without getting blocked in your body as excess fat.

- The leaves of the Moringa plant are rich in fiber, which is needed by the body for the digestive system to function properly. Fiber helps the body to get rid of the excess food that is not needed for a healthy body.

- Fiber, which is found in abundance in Moringa leaves, also act to sate hunger so that you get hungry less as well as less often. This is a big help if you are on a diet or trying to skip overeating.

- Moringa leaves are also one of the most low-calorie food available in nature, but one that also has every other nutrition element needed in the body. If you are a person who can never stick to a diet because you feel hungry and not sated, then Moringa leaves are the perfect answer for you.

Since these leaves are extremely low on calories, eating a huge amount of them are not harmful to your health or to your diet. You can eat all the Moringa leaves that you want, and not gain any extra wealth. At the same time, you won't be missing out on any other nutrition because the leaves have them all.

However, all these weight loss benefits of Moringa could be achieved only through eating a large amount of leaves all day, every day, for a long period of time. Especially if you are overweight or looking forward to losing a huge amount of weight, this could mean months of eating nothing more than Moringa leaves, which could slowly become dreary and revolting.

This could mean giving up on the diet of Moringa before you even achieve the goal. Therefore, what we need is a more subtle yet more definitive introduction of Moringa Oleifera into our daily diets, so that nothing changes much in our lifestyles.

That can be achieved with some other products that also originate from the Moringa plant, such as powdered Moringa leaves, or tea made from Moringa leaf. Also, the seeds from the Moringa pods are also effective in helping a person to lose weight.

MORINGA LEAF POWDER

Moringa leaves are made into powder after being shade dried and crushed. This powder can be used in cooking any dish, or drank directly mixed with any drink. Consuming this powder regularly, in limited amount, along with any normal and low-calorie, low-carbohydrate and low-fat diet will definitely prove to be effective.

This is especially effective for people who, for various reasons, fail to lose weight even when they are constantly on severe diets and do not overeat.

MORINGA LEAF TEA

Moringa tea is made by boiling the leaves of the Moringa plant in water for a few minutes. The tea that is prepared from these leaves help in losing weight by increasing the metabolism rate of the body and helping digestion.

Drinking Moringa leaf tea instead of your regular caffeine at least once or twice a day will certainly assist you in your weight loss journey.

MORINGA SEEDS

Moringa seeds are also, if taken in limits ever day, are effective for weight loss techniques. However, these seeds are concentrated with a huge amount of nutrients and should not be taken a lot.

For a healthy adult who wants to lose weight, as many as 4 to 5 Moringa seeds per day are more than enough to start your routine with. If you want to lose weight fast and decide to take more than 10 Moringa seeds everyday for a faster result, it may actually have an adverse effect on you and you may start losing 'too much' weight 'too fast' - something that is not healthy, however desirable.

Not all the people who are overweight and obese are overeaters or people who cannot diet or exercise. Many of them are obese because they suffer from a bad metabolism, i.e. they have trouble digesting and passing on food.

Moringa Oleifera is an extremely effective way to develop your existing metabolism system so that the food that you eat can be easily digested and does not stay behind in your body in the form of love handles and guts.

Also, consuming Moringa regularly - either in the form of powder or tea - gives your body energy. Not the type of short-lived energy that we get after consuming sugar or carbohydrate, but the more lasting energy that will help us live an active life and exercise.

Therefore, as we can see, the different parts of the Moringa Oleifera plant may not actually and directly help a person shed all their unwanted and excess weight fast and straight, but it is an effective way of complementing your existing diet. It is also an excellent lifestyle choice in order to maintain a healthy and happy life.

V. MORINGA: DETOXIFICATION POSSIBILITIES

Detoxification is another concept that has become very important to many people, at least in the recent year, since its importance in health was first established.

As we mentioned at the very first few paragraphs on this book, our modern-day diets and eating habits are extremely unhealthy and harmful. We seem to be living on a diet of processed and packaged food, unnecessary fats and carbohydrates, alcohol and other harmful food and drink that may be giving us pleasure but slowly adding harmful toxins into our body.

LIVER DISEASE AND DETOXIFICATION

The function of the liver in our body is to detoxify all the harmful things that enter our body; its main responsibility is to separate the toxins from the food and drinks that we consume and keep our body and the other organs safe from them. The food and drinks - even the air that we breathe in - are filled with different types of harmful toxins that we are regularly putting in us. As a result, our livers are exhausted fighting with these toxins and we face various diseases and conditions that mainly affect the liver.

Our exhausted liver, therefore, faces many problems and eventually results in diseases of the liver. This leads to Cirrhosis or scarring of the liver tissues, and ultimately, liver failure.

Two of the main causes of Cirrhosis and Liver Failure are alcohol abuse and the accumulation of fat on the liver due to overconsumption of non-alcoholic fat.

Other causes of Liver Diseases include:

- Hepatitis A, B & C

- Autoimmune Hepatitis

- Sclerosing cholangitis

- Biliary Cirrhosis

- Wilson's Disease

- Hemochromatosis

- Hyperoxaluria & Oxalosis

- Liver Cancer & Liver Adenoma, and

- Bile Duct Cancer.

Besides, liver diseases are also caused by intake of:

- ethyl alcohol (in the drinking alcohols),

- peroxide (mainly from the per oxidized oils that we consume),

- Aflatoxins (toxins in our food),

- Pharmaceuticals (from the antibiotics that we take),

- Chemotherapies (for cancer), and

- Environmental Pollutants (pollution in the air, water and soil).

Together, these chemicals are known as hepatotoxic chemicals. The more we take in these hepatotoxic chemicals through various mediums, as listed above, the more the liver is affected and loses its capability of detoxifying our bodies.

Moringa Oleifera has been diagnosed with having properties

that fight these hepatotoxic chemicals. It can, through proper use, help restore the affected liver to its original and working condition.

However, please note that it is not actually possible for Moringa to cure any advanced cases of liver disease. Taking Moringa can detoxify the liver of any residue of hepatotoxic chemicals and reverse some of the harms done to the liver, but it cannot cure a long-time illness that has been caused by long time abuse of hepatotoxic chemicals.

Also, if you are looking forward to detoxifying your liver through Moringa, it's better to do it properly and totally; i.e. without cramming our body with other toxic pollutants and alcoholic substances while, at the same time, attempting detoxification. While the liver is in the process of being detoxified with Moringa Oleifera plant, our main diet should also be pure, simple and healthy.

MORINGA TEA AND DETOXIFICATION

Moringa tea - i.e. the tea made by boiling the green Moringa leaves in water - has been used in traditional medicine for centuries as a method of cleansing and detoxifying the body. Drinking this tea regularly - together with the aid of a balanced and healthy diet - can definitely help in removing all the signs of toxins from our body, slowly but entirely.

Research into the Moringa Oleifera tea has shown many ways through which it can effectively cure many liver disorders by removing harmful toxins. We will discuss this in later chapters of this book.

MORINGA AND OVERALL DETOXIFICATION OF THE BODY

An overall detoxification of the whole body, especially the liver, has been seen in people who are regular consumers of Moringa - either of the leaves as vegetables, the seeds, Moringa flowers, pods, or Moringa tea.

From various researches conducted on the affects of the Moringa plant, it has been known to aid in detoxification in the following ways:

- The different elements of the Moringa plant assists in the elimination of harmful and toxic metal from the body that is more than the normal range.

- Moringa completely prevents the mitochondrial changes in the body that are caused by ethanol.

- Moringa motivates the arrangement of the metal-binding proteins that detoxify the metals present inside the human body, especially the liver.

- Moringa, in some cases and in some parts, counteracts the damage caused by excessive alcohol consumption.

Thus, it can be seen that, taken regularly and in limits, the Moringa Oleifera certainly has been proved to be effective in detoxifying the body of harmful toxins and pollutants.

VI. MORINGA: OTHER USES AND APPLICATIONS

By now, we have learned quite enough of how Moringa is used in cooking, eating, health, beauty and skincare. However, there are some other surprising uses of the Moringa Oleifera that are not so widely known but are still very important in certain localities of the world.

MORINGA SEEDCAKE AND WATER PURIFICATION

One such use of Moringa is in purifying water, i.e. water treatment. In many West African countries, the seeds of the Moringa plants - after the oil has been extracted - are used to detoxify and purify water for drinking.

The oil that is extracted from the seeds found inside the pods (fruits) of the Moringa tree are used in a number of beauty, hair and skin products as well as for consumption. However, the seed cake, i.e. the substance that remains after the oil has been extracted, has further important use to mankind.

The seed-cake, substances that are white and papery around the crushed seed, contains flocculating properties that are a sustainable source of water purification, as opposed to other chemical methods which include soda ash and aluminum sulphate. Moreover, this is an affordable method compared to other such ways of purifying water that is also easily available in rural areas.

Almost all rural communities of Africa use Moringa seedcake to purify their drinking water on a household basis. It is also possible to use this procedure on a large scale; many studies are being conducted to make that possibility come true.

MORINGA LEAVES FOR POULTRY FARMING

Poultry is an important source of income, a profession and also an important source of nutrition in many developing and underdeveloped countries in the world, especially in the African and Asian countries. In many of these regions, Moringa Oleifera leaves play a significant part as food for animals, mainly chicken.

Other traditional feed for chicken in poultry farming included fishmeal and other leaf meals - all of which are expensive and cost up to 60% to 80% of the total cost raising chicken. Moreover, these chicken feeds are not always available and require to be bought from stores or additional cultivation of fish.

Moringa leaves, on the other hand, are an excellent source of protein and other necessary minerals, vitamins and oxycaretenoids. They are also available for growing in any rural areas; moreover, they are actually grown in many households because of their nutritional and medicinal values and are available at hand.

MORINGA LEAVES FOR CATTLE FARMING

Moringa leaves are also used as feed for beef and milk cows as well as for swine. It has been noticed that by when Moringa leaves constitute 50% of the daily nutrition for cows, their milk production and overall weight increases by more than 30%.

However, Moringa leaves should not be the only feed given to cattle; rather it should be balanced with molasses, young sorghum plants and sugarcane. If the daily feed of cattle consists of a ratio of Moringa leaves that is more than 50% of the total feed, it would result in excess fat production in them. This could be fatal in cattle farming.

MORINGA LEAVES AS ANIMAL FOOD

Beside chicken and cattle farming, Moringa leaves can also be fed to other animals, i.e. goats, sheep, rabbits and pigs. These animals actually enjoy the taste of these leaves and it also helps in increasing their weight and their nutrition.

A daily feed that consists of 50% Moringa leaves and 50% other elements, such as maize, Leucaena and salt will ensure a significant growth rate in pigs at very little cost.

In rabbits, a daily meal of crushed or processed Moringa leaves could lead to noteworthy weight gain and digestibility. It can also help in lowering blood pressure in rabbits and can be used as their fractional or entire source of protein.

MORINGA SOAP FOR CLEANING PURPOSES

The leaves of the Moringa tree can also be made into soaps as they contain strong and influential anti-bacterial elements. This is not yet a popular use of the Moringa plant, even in rural areas where Moringa plays a significant role in many other aspects. May tests and research is being done to enhance this side of the Moringa plant so that it can be used as a sustainable method of cleanliness.

Moringa leaves can be crushed and blended to make into a soap which can be used in washing hand, and in general cleanliness.

We will discuss this in details further in the chapter of this book which deals with the medicinal properties of Moringa. This soap made from Moringa leaves have been known to sterilize *E. Coli* and other such dangerous germs from the human body.

MORINGA SEEDS AS BIO-FUEL

In very recent years, it has been seen that Moringa seeds can be used as alternative sources of fuel that will be economical as well as environmentally efficient.

The seeds of the Moringa plant are constituted of 35% to 40% oil. This oil can be extracted in a number of ways, and the oil can be used in many skin and hair care products as well as for consumption. However, in some households, this oil is used as as biodiesel for cooking purposes.

Ongoing research shows good possibilities of using Moringa oil and seeds as biodiesel in the future. However, much more research is needed on this topic to guarantee this hypothesis.

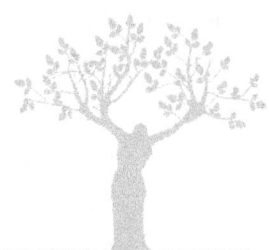

Chapter 3

NUTRITIONAL VALUES OF MORINGA

There is almost no limit to the benefits and usefulness of the *Moringa Oleifera* plant in human life. We would require an extremely long chapter to describe all the benefits of this super food.

While most plants, fruits and vegetables are good in one or two nutritional categories, this plant has almost every type of nutrition that is necessary in the human body, including some of the rare ones that is found in very few other vegetations. Almost all parts of this wondrous plant can be used in our lives in a variety of needs.

We will start with the nutritional value we can get by consuming *Moringa Oleifera*.

Mainly, the leaves and roots of the Moringa plant are consumed as food. In some regions, the flowers and the pods are also eaten as food.

MORINGA LEAVES

The leaves of the Moringa tree are the most nutritional part of the tree, and are an excellent source of essential iron, calcium, Protein, Manganese, Vitamin A and B, and Vitamin C.

The leaves are boiled in water and eaten like spinach; however, this is not an effective recipe because most of the nutrition is washed way with the water that is thrown away after boiling. The more common practice is to shade dry the leaves and crush them into a powder, to be used as a condiment or supplement in cooking any dish. However, excessive heating while cooking may also decrease the nutrition.

Moringa Leaves contain the following nutrition in abundance:

- Calcium, which is needed for strong bones and teeth,

- Protein, which builds the body and the muscles,

- Potassium, which develops the brain and the power of thinking,

- Manganese, which is important for metabolism and the antioxidant system,

- Beta-carotene, which reduces the risk of breast cancer in women,

- Vitamin A, which helps in preventing diseases of the eyes, skin, heart and stomach

- Vitamin B, which helps in cell metabolism, and

- Vitamin C, which fights flu and the common cold.

If you are still not convinced, see below the nutritional

properties that can be found in just 100gm (5 cups) of raw and sun-dried Moringa leaf powder.

Energy	64 kcal
Fat	1.40 gm
Protein	9.40 gm
Carbohydrates	8.28 gm
Dietary Fiber	2.0 gm
Vitamins	
- Vitamin A	378 micro gm
- Vitamin B1 (Thiamine)	0.257 mg
- Vitamin B1 (Riboflavin)	0.660 mg
- Vitamin B3 (Niacin)	2.220 mg
- Vitamin B5 (Pantothenic)	0.125 mg
- Vitamin B6	1.200 mg
- Vitamin B9 (Folate)	40 micro gm
Vitamin C	51.7 mg
Calcium	185 mg
Iron	4.0 mg
Magnesium	147 mg
Manganese	0.36 mg
Potassium	337 mg
Sodium	9 mg
Zinc	0.06 mg

Phosphorus   112mg

Water   78.66 mg

– Source: Wikipedia.com

Besides, Moringa leaves also contain some rare nutrition, such as:

- 92 types of nutrients,

- 46 types of antioxidants,

- 18 types of amino acids and 9 essential amino acids, and

- 36 types of anti-inflammatory

To enhance the nutritional properties of Moringa in a more common language, we can say that raw powdered Moringa leaves has:

- 4 times the Vitamin A found in Carrots,

- 7 times the Vitamin C found in Oranges,

- 2 times the Protein of Yogurt,

- 3 times the Iron found in Almonds,

- 3 times the Potassium of Bananas and

- 4 times the Calcium of Pure Cow Milk.

In a single serving of raw or dried Moringa leaves, you will be able to fulfill

- 71% of your daily Iron needs

- 125% of your daily Calcium needs

- 41% of your daily Potassium needs

- 61% of your daily Magnesium needs

- 272% of your daily vitamin A needs

- 22% of your daily Vitamin C needs

The leaves may be the most diversely nutritious part of the plant, but it is not the only useful part of it.

MORINGA PODS

The green, young and immature seed pods of Moringa are usually consumed as food in the Asian regions and commonly known as 'drumsticks' because of the way they look. They are cut up and cooked as vegetables; the vitamins stay intact inside the pods even after being cooked over high fire.

Moringa pods are generally eaten when they are raw and soft. They are delicious when cooked and eaten as curry and soup.

Green Moringa pods are highly enriched in potassium, manganese, dietary fiber and magnesium, among other nutrients. The complete list is given below for 100 gm of raw and green Moringa pods:

Energy	37 kcal
Fat	2.20 gm
Protein	2.10 gm
Carbohydrates	8.53 gm
Dietary Fiber	3.2 gm
Vitamins	
- Vitamin A	4 micro gm

- Vitamin B1 (Thiamine)	0.053 mg
- Vitamin B1 (Riboflavin)	0.074 mg
- Vitamin B3 (Niacin)	0.620 mg
- Vitamin B6	0.120 mg
-Vitamin B9 (Folate)	44 micro gm
Vitamin C	141.0 mg
Calcium	30 mg
Iron	0.36 mg
Magnesium	45 mg
Manganese	0.259 mg
Potassium	461 mg
Sodium	42 mg
Zinc	0.045 mg
Phosphorus	50 mg
Water	88.20 mg

– Source: Wikipedia.com

When the pods become mature, they are broken in for their seeds, which are used for a lot of other reasons.

MORINGA SEEDS

Seeds are obtained from mature Moringa pods when they are brown and hard. The seeds, too, are an unusual source of nutrition.

The seeds can be eaten directly when they are raw inside the mature pods and contain high amounts of amino acids, minerals, proteins and vitamins in a concentrated form. The oil that is extracted from the seeds is also rich in nourishment and used for many purposes.

MORINGA ROOTS AND BARKS

Almost all the nutritional properties that are found in all the other parts of the Moringa tree are also found in the roots, more concentrated. The roots and barks of this tree have a sharp and tangy taste and contain polyphenols.

They are used to make a special sauce which is considered a culinary treat in many regions and contains high fiber, minerals, vitamins and proteins.

MORINGA FLOWERS

Moringa flowers contain vital amino acids, potassium and calcium that are needed in the body.

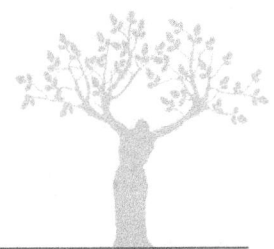

Chapter 4

MEDICINAL PROPERTIES OF MORINGA

Besides being used as food and condiment for cooking, the different parts of the plant are also used as medicines to help prevent diseases as well as provide easing from various illnesses and ailments.

MORINGA ROOTS

- Moringa roots have been used in the ancient practices of Ayurveda since a long time, and acknowledged for its wonderful medicinal properties in being able to treat a number of ailments.

- Moringa roots were used in traditional Indian medicine to control different cardiovascular diseases.

- The intake of these roots, in small doses, has been known to help with Irritable Bowel Syndrome, upset stomach and other gastric-related discomforts.

- Poultices made with Moringa roots helps in easing arthritis pain and cramps. This can be also used be used in backaches, rheumatism and kidney pain.

- Moringa roots are used as tonic for skin inflammation.

- Moringa roots, taken in careful and small doses, can enhance appetite and help in keeping the digestive tracts clear.

- Roots of the Moringa plant show great results in reducing swelling and in healing edema.

- Moringa root have been used to treat impotence and sexual dysfunction in ancient times.

- Extracts from Moringa roots have help in eliminating kidney stones by flushing out phosphate and calcium from the kidney.

- Moringa roots contain rare elements and nutrients that help the body combat ovarian cancer, as well as help cancer patients.

- Moringa roots extracts can be considered an important pharmaceutical supplementary, as it can trigger better sleep in patients who are taking powerful pain medications.

- Moringa Roots can be used as a laxative for constipation.

- Moringa roots also works well as antiseptics and can be used topically for any problems in the skin.

However, all the elements that are found in the roots of the Moringa tree are concentrated and extremely powerful compared to the other parts of the plant, and should therefore be applied or consumed in small doses.

EXPERIMENTS WITH MORINGA ROOT EXTRACTS

In many of the developing countries of the world, diarrhea is a major problem, especially in cases of children under the age of five. Around the world, more than 8 million children die of diarrhea each year.

In ancient Indian medicine, Moringa root extracts have played a significant role in the cure of severe diarrhea. Therefore, at the *C. K. Pithawala institute of Pharmaceutical Sciences and Research, Gujrat, India,* in 2010, a very important experiment was undertaken to test the effects of this miraculous root on severe cases of diarrhea in rats. Rats were chosen in this experiment as their biological and their genetic characteristics, as well as their behaviors, resemble very closely to that of humans.

30 rats were divided into five groups, and were induced to diarrhea by injecting castor oil. One group received saline as cure, the second group received atropine; the other three groups received various doses of Moringa Oleifera root extract. The results showed that that intensity of diarrhea was reduced by 47.67%, 56.25% and 61.74% in the three groups that received the different doses of this root extract compared to the group that received saline water. On the other hand, the result was only a reduction of 33.38% for the group that received atropine.

It can be successfully deducted from this experiment that the root extracts of the Moringa Oleifera plant can actually help cure, or at least reduce, the severity of diarrhea in people. The details of this experiment can be found here.

MORINGA LEAVES

Moringa leaves are rich in anti-bacterial and anti-inflammatory properties, and can thus be very helpful in treating minor cuts, bruises and wounds, as well as insect bites.

Moringa leaves are known to work as first aid on shallow cuts and to stop bleeding. They are also helpful in reducing diarrhea. Moringa leaves cure fever, bronchitis and give relief in eye and ear infection; these leaves also treat inflammation of the mucus membrane.

However, one of the most important roles of the leaf extracts of the Moringa plant are its therapeutic properties that work against severe liver injury.

EXPERIMENTS WITH MORINGA LEAF EXTRACTS

An experiment conducted at the *University Colleges of Science and Technology, University of Calcutta, India,* in 2012 proved that application of Moringa leaf extracts help in preventing liver injury in mice that has been fed a high-fat diet.

In this experiment, a group of mice were fed a High-fat Diet (HFD) which could lead to Non-Alcoholic Fatty Liver Disease (NAFLD), and ultimately to other more serious ailments. The mice were also injected with a low dose of *Moringa Oleifera Leaf Extract* (MOLF), which showed a significant reduction to the injuries in the liver caused by the HFD. At the same time, the introduction of MOLF to the mice also showed reduction in the earlier signs of fatty liver that were caused before the induction of the HFD.

Therefore it can be said that extracts of the Moringa leaf has both preventive as well as curative properties that work on an injured liver. The details of the experiment can be found here.

Another experiment was conducted at the *Tel-Aviv Sourasky Medical Center, Tel-Aviv, Israel* in 2013 that concluded that the aqueous leaf extracts of the Moringa plant increases the cytotoxic effects of chemotherapy given for pancreatic cancer.

Fewer than 6% of the patients suffering from pancreatic cancer survive more than 6/7 years, even after regular chemotherapy sessions. This study was conducted to find the effects of the Moringa leaf extracts on the pancreatic cancer cells, namely Panc-1, p34, and COLO 357. The question was whether the extracts would increase the cytotoxic effects of chemotherapy or reduce the cancer cells' resistance to the chemotherapy.

The result of the experiment showed that the Moringa leaf extracts have inhibited the growth of all the pancreatic cells; it also significantly increased the efficiency of the cytotoxic effect of the chemotherapy session on the human pancreatic cancer cells.

The details of this experiment can be found here.

MORINGA PODS

Raw Moringa pods are eaten as a de-warmer to treat spleen and liver problems. It is also known for its anti-oxidant and anti-diabetic effects in treating diabetes.

EXPERIMENTS WITH MORINGA PODS

At the Centre for Advanced Studies, Department of Zoology, University of Rajasthan, India, in 2011, an experiment was conducted to evaluate the anti-oxidant and anti-diabetic properties of Moringa Pods in experimental diabetes, i.e. on Streptozotocin (STZ) induced diabetic rats.

These rats were artificially induced to Diabetes and then treated with Moringa Oleifera pods (MOMtE). The results were measured by the changes in their biochemical parameters, both in their serum and in their pancreatic tissue. After 21 days, significant reduction was seen in serum glucose and nitric oxide. Also, the treatment with MOMtE showed increased levels of antioxidant in the pancreatic tissue.

It was concluded that, MOMtE exerts significant protective effects against STZ-induced diabetes and exhibits significant anti-diabetic and anti-oxidant activity. The details of the experiment can be found here.

MORINGA SEEDS

Moringa Seeds contain antibiotic and fungicide Terygospermin, and is an effective treatment against the skin-infecting bacteria, namely Staphylococcus Aureus, and Pseudomonas Aeruginosa.

Moreover, Moringa seeds are also known for their anti-inflammatory and anti-oxidant properties that can have beneficial effects on colitis, which is an inflammation of the inner lining of the colon.

EXPERIMENTS WITH MORINGA SEEDS

An experiment was conducted to test the anti-inflammatory effects of Moringa seeds on acute acetic colitis of rats at the Isfahan Pharmaceutical Sciences Research Center, I. R. Iran, in 2014. The main goal of this experiment was to see whether the anti-colitis elements present in these seeds are beneficial to the inflammation caused by colitis.

Hydro-alcoholic extract (MSHE) and the chloroform fraction (MCF) of the Moringa seeds were given orally to separate groups of male rats who were induced to acute colitis. This was continued for 5 days, during which Prednisolone and normal saline were also given to the rats. 24 hours after the last dose, the tissue injuries of the rats were assessed, both macroscopically and pathologically.

It was seen that the doses of MSHE and MCF were able to reduce the severity and area of the ulcer as well as the inflammation in the mucus membrane, the severity and extent of the crypt damage, and the parameters of colitis.

It could be concluded from the experiment that both MSHE and MCF found in Moringa seeds were able to reduce severity in colitis. The details of this experiment can be found here.

MORINGA SEED OIL

Moringa seed Oil - or as it is also known as, Behen Oil, or Ben Oil - is also known to be used in the treatment of scurvy, hysteria and prostate problems.

Moringa plant parts have been used in ancient Ayurveda and Siddha medicine for thousands of years. It is only in the last few decades that the modern world has rediscovered the benefits of this miracle tree that could solve a lot of the medical problems that we have.

The various parts of the Moringa Oleifera plant have other many medicinal benefits that are continuously being experimented and researched on. The experiments and tests mentioned in this chapter were only but a few of the hundred others that are being conducted everyday all over the world. Scientist, doctors and nutritionists are trying to find other uses of the Moringa Oleifera plant that can help us battle and cure many more serious diseases that we face in our modern worlds.

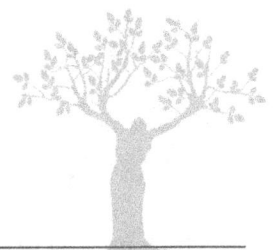

Chapter 5

THE ROLE OF MORINGA IN POVERTY AND DEVELOPMENT

Although Moringa Oleifera grows in many developing and underdeveloped countries of Asia and Africa, its use was limited and could not reach its full potential in most of these areas. In many of them, the natives of the countries where Moringa grows in abundance only know it as a vegetable that they eat regularly, unaware of its potential contribution to other aspects of their lives - health, beauty and nutrition.

In many households around the world, Moringa leaves and pods are cooked in a way that greatly diminishes their extraordinary nutritional value, leaving the residue dish nothing more than a mildly nutritious vegetable. Besides, the leaves, flowers and the seeds of the Moringa tea are used, in some areas, as cure for simple day-to-day elements such as the common cold, cramps, headache and backache, without realizing the true potential and the reach of this plant in medical science.

However, Moringa is actually a recent find in modern science and it is only in the last few years that scientists have noticed this plant and its astonishing promise, thus naming it the 'miracle tree'. Slowly and gradually, knowledge and breeding of this tree is spreading across the world as a medium of nutrition, health, beauty as well as for detoxification and weight loss purposes.

MORINGA AROUND THE WORLD

In a number of countries across the globe, Moringa Oleifera is making an appearance in the daily diet and lifestyle of thousands of households. Thanks to the awareness and help of a few organizations - to be more specific, Trees for Life International, The World Church Service, the Christian and Missionary Alliance, the Educational Concerns for Hunger Organization and the Volunteer Partnerships for West Africa - millions of people all around the world are finally recognizing this wonderful plant that can do so much for mankind.

In **Haiti,** one of the poorest countries of the world, more than 30% children of the total population is chronically malnourished and at severe risk. Very recently, Moringa Oleifera plants has been rediscovered growing locally in Haiti, forgotten for generations. After the earthquake of 2010 and the hurricanes of 2012, Haiti is hopeful of the aid of this miracle plant for the reconstruction of their country, in numerous ways, i.e. as their main source of nutrition, and as first aid and medicine for a number of ailments, especially for the children of Haiti.

The Moringa plants, with its large disposition, is being used to provide shade for their production of coffee beans - which incidentally happens to be the main source of income for more than 100,000 households across the country. The leaves of this tree are also being used as animal feed for cattle, poultry and fish rearing.

In rural **Zimbabwe**, Moringa Oleifera grows in the backyard of every household, and contributes to the family's nutrition, health, animal feed and income. It has enabled all these families to become self sufficient on a sustainable basis.

In **Malawi**, the demand for soya bean oil had always been greater than their national production, and had been imported from South America. However, with the advent of the Moringa plant, Malawi has not only become self-sufficient in oil production enough for cooking and other purposes, but has also found a new source of income.

USES OF MORINGA IN DEVELOPING COUNTRIES

It is needless to say that the benefits of the Moringa Oleifera plant would be more effective in the developing and the underdeveloped countries of the world rather than the countries which are already self-sufficient and adequate. There are multiple aspects where Moringa can be used in these regions.

One of the most important problems of underdeveloped and developing countries of the world is malnutrition, especially in children. According to FAO, the total number of malnourished people in the world in 2011 was 925 million. Congo, Eritrea, Burundi, Haiti and Sierra Leone were the top 5 countries where malnutrition is most serious.

Moringa is the perfect solution to malnutrition in most of these countries. It is an inexpensive plant that grows locally in many countries of the world, doesn't need much care or incentive, but can provide multiple times the necessary nutrients that the human body needs. By including Moringa leaves, fruits and flowers in their everyday diet, the inhabitants of these developing countries can fulfill almost all their dietary needs in 2/3 servings per day.

More than 670,000 children die around the world annually due to Vitamin A insufficiency, a nutrient that is found in carrots. However, carrots are relatively expensive and do not grow in many regions of the world where it is needed the most. Moringa leaves, on the other hand, contains 4 times the Vitamin A present in carrots and are more accessible.

According to WHO, more than 9 million children, under the age of five, die every year due to malnutrition. These children do not have access to nutritious food from when they are born. Their mothers, being malnourished themselves, are not able to provide them with enough breast milk to sustain their health. Elements in the Moringa Oleifera plant leaves help increase the quantity as well as the quality of breast milk in mothers so that these children get a better start in life.

In **Cambodia**, 66% of all pregnant women are anemic, and lead to a high child and mother mortality rate. The main cause of this is the lack of iron - a deficiency which can be easily solved with Moringa leaves which contains 3 times the Iron found in almonds.

Access to safe and clean drinking water is also one of the main problems that many backward countries face, and it is also one of the reasons behind diarrhea, dehydration and other bacteria-related diseases. The seeds of the Moringa plant, as it have been found out quite recently, could be used to purify waters from wells, lakes, rivers and even from rain. It is also extremely inexpensive, easily available and easy to use.

Besides, the leaves and the pods of the Moringa plant is

also used to treat severe diarrhea, cold and flu, rheumatism and migraine pains, as well as providing nutrition to the population of the remote areas where modern medicines are not available.

For these reasons, organizations like UNDP, FAO and UNICEF are working relentlessly to spread awareness of this miracle tree so that every household in every rural locality of these countries, and many others, become self-sufficient in providing nutrition and basic medical attention to themselves.

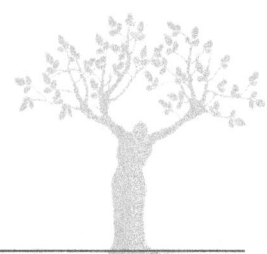

Chapter 6

MORINGA: WARNINGS AND SIDE EFFECTS

*M*oringa Oleifera is known as the 'Miracle tree' because it has a miraculous and positive effect on almost every aspect of our lives. However, there are some limitations to using Moringa, especially in the amount that it can be taken.

Like all other good things in life, Moringa Oleifera should also be taken in limits. One should always know of the warning signs of using Moringa before using this plant in their daily lives.

Some of the parts of the Moringa plant are extremely concentrated, namely the roots and the seeds. So, special caution must be taken when it comes to consuming these parts of the plant. The other parts of the plant, i.e. the leaves, the flowers and the pods (fruits) are relatively harmless and can be consumed or used in any form preferred. Only the roots and the seeds need to be carefully handled as they are unusually concentrated in nutrients and contain many elements which may prove to be severe if taken directly and without thoughts of any consequences.

If you are thinking on including Moringa Oleifera in your life and in your daily diet, do keep the following tips and warnings in mind.

#1. DO NOT EAT MORINGA SEEDS IF YOU ARE PREGNANT!

If you are pregnant, or suspect that you are pregnant, **IMMEDIATELY STOP** eating Moringa seeds. This also includes the roots and the barks of the Moringa plant. These parts of the plant contain certain elements that can make the uterus contract; this can lead to miscarriage and premature labor.

However, other parts of the Moringa plant, i.e. the leaves and the powder, can be consumed in limited amounts. They are actually beneficial to both the child and the mother during and after pregnancy.

This is often a tricky situation to solve, because many women use Moringa seeds to lose weight or as an aphrodisiac to increase their sex drive - as both factors are somewhat connected to conceiving. Therefore, it is very important to know the exact limit between when you are trying to get pregnant and when you are actually pregnant. You should stop taking Moringa seeds and roots immediately if you think you have conceived, no questions asked.

#2. DO NOT EAT MORINGA SEEDS IF YOU ARE TRYING TO CONCEIVE!

If you are looking to conceive, then Moringa seeds, roots and barks are also a big 'no-no' for you.

This is another tricky situation because the leaves of the Moringa plant are very useful in increasing libido and sex drive. However, if you are - at the same time - trying to conceive, you must not take Moringa seeds as they are a natural method of birth control.

In rural India, many women take Moringa seeds and roots regularly as a natural way to prevent pregnancy. It is an extremely inexpensive and natural, and doesn't affect the body negatively or create any long-term problems with fertility.

#3. DO NOT EAT MORINGA SEEDS IF YOU ARE BREASTFEEDING!

Another huge dilemma and another paradox that we have here with Moringa seeds verses Moringa leaves when it comes to lactating and breastfeeding mothers. Moringa leaves and leaf powder facilitate and increase the amount and quality of breast milk in mothers that is extremely beneficial to infants and toddlers.

At the same time, the effects of Moringa seeds - also the roots and barks - are still undetermined and are suspected to be harmful when passed to the children through breastfeeding.

Research is still going on regarding whether Moringa seeds and roots actually affect the children much, but in the meantime, it is safer to avoid these parts of the plant and stick to the leaves and leaf powder.

#4. DO NOT EAT MORE THAN 5 MORINGA SEEDS IN A DAY!

That is the estimated limit of Moringa seeds that can be consumed in a single day - 5 (five)! Any healthy and willing adult can take up to 5 (five) Moringa seeds a day, and not more than that, and not more than 2 (two) at one time.

Since the Moringa seeds are extremely concentrated, they have a very strong effect on the human body, which includes an upset stomach, nausea, dizziness, or even severe food poisoning. Since Moringa seeds are usually taken for weight loss purposes, some people tend to consume a large number of seeds at once for rapid weight loss - something which would definitely prove to be harmful for their body.

However, these seeds affect different people in different ways. For some, the effects may be less than others; while some people feel sick after only consuming 2 (two) Moringa seeds at one time, others may easily digest up to 10 (ten).

Therefore, it is important that you start small - with 1 (one) seed the first few day; then 2 (two), and then increase the total consumption to 4 (four) or 5 (five) seeds per day. This way, your body will slowly get used to Moringa seeds.

#5. DO NOT EAT MORINGA SEEDS WHEN YOUR STOMACH IS EMPTY!

Moringa seeds are not supposed to be eaten when you are hungry or when your stomach is empty. Eating these seeds on an empty stomach - no matter how few you consumed - will definitely result in vomiting, dizziness and ultimately, in purging.

Moringa seeds should be taken in limited amounts after a big meal, and as a snack.

#6. DO NOT EAT MORINGA SEEDS WITHOUT PEELING!

Moringa seeds are not supposed to be eaten with the peels still on; this is not the hygienic procedure. Always remove the peel, and clean the Moringa seeds adequately with warm water and salt before eating them.

Although, people who are looking forward to losing weight via Moringa seeds usually eat them with the peel on. This is because Moringa seed peels are extremely fibrous and facilitate fast weight loss. However, this is neither hygienic, nor recommended.

Some other side effects, though not too serious, of Moringa may be:

- **Nausea**. If you are new to Moringa, you might experience some nausea after the first few times. This is especially an indication that you are probably taking too much Moringa than needed, or than your body is used to. The best strategy would be to slowly introduce Moringa into your body and into your diet plan instead of abruptly.

- **Diarrhea**. Moringa is a powerful laxative, especially the powdered Moringa leaves. Many people who suffer from constipation take Moringa powder for cleansing their stomach. However, since it is a powerful laxative, taking too much Moringa could lead to severe diarrhea and frequent trips to the washroom.

- **Heartburn**. Straight intake of Moringa, such as, Moringa powder mixed with water and drank, or Moringa seeds taken directly, may cause heartburn. If this is the case with you, perhaps it is best that you consume Moringa cooking it as a vegetable, or adding the powder to your cooked meals for the nutrition.

- **Blood Thickening**. Moringa has properties that thicken the blood when consumed as food. So if you are on blood thinning medicines for some reason, it is better to stop taking Moringa - in any form, but especially the seeds and the roots. Consult a doctor if you want to include Moringa in your lifestyle for added nutrition when on blood-thinning medications.

- **Blood disorders**. In a few special cases, the use of Moringa seeds have shown signs of blood disorders, such as increase in the count of white blood cells, lower amount of blood platelets, petechiae or bleeding in the gums. Though rare, these situations could lead to something more serious. It is, therefore, better to consult a doctor before trying out Moringa seeds if you have any issues with your blood.

- **Gag Reflex**. Moringa has a very distinct and spicy taste, and can cause a gag reflex in some people, which could lead to temporary loss of appetite and nausea. If this is the case, it would be better not to try to consume Moringa directly as powder, seeds or tea, but to include them in cooked and baked meals.

After all these warnings and side effects, the positive achievements of Moringa outweigh everything else. This is something that should definitely be introduced into our lifestyles. However, we will leave this chapter with some final words of warning.

- Go slow in introducing Moringa - any part of it - into your lifestyle and into your diet. There's no hurry about it. Make it a slow but sustainable prologue into your life, and keep it in it.

- Always exercise caution when it comes to the intake of the roots, barks, and the seeds of the Moringa plant. Consult a doctor if you suffer from any side effects, or if you are confused about a particular health problem before consuming these parts of the Moringa plant.

- Remember: Too much of everything is bad, even when it is something as 'good' and 'beneficial' as Moringa. Don't take too much of it, whatever your reasons are. Even if you are looking for rapid weight loss with Moringa seeds, control yourself so that you do not exceed the average limit. Even losing too much weight too fast is harmful for you.

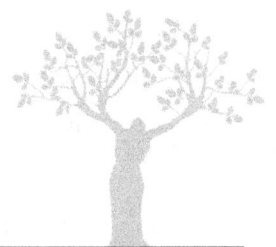

Chapter 7

MORINGA (RECIPES, BEAUTY AND OTHER PREPARATIONS)

U p till now, we have been learning about all the goodness of the Moringa Oleifera plant, and how it can positively affect our health, nutrition, beauty and lifestyle. In this chapter, we would go further into the topic and learn how to prepare and introduce Moringa into our lives, with some easy and simple recipes that would be effortless to introduce into our daily meals.

We would also learn some other interesting techniques of preparing health and beauty products using Moringa, namely Moringa facial masks and creams, Moringa soap and other similar cleanliness products.

MORINGA HEALTHY RECIPES

We will share with you some undemanding recipes using the different parts of the Moringa plant that would not be too alien to your unaccustomed taste buds but would ensure maximum nutrition and effect.

i. Moringa Leaf Tea

For Moringa Tea, you will leave 4/5 stalks of mature leaves. It is better to use the mature leaves as they dry up faster than the young green leaves.

Dry the leaves (along with the stalks) in natural environment for a few days. Do not dry them under the sun, as that will diminish the nutrition inside the leaves. When the leaves and the stalks are dry, grind them up roughly in a spice grinder. You can completely crush the leaves into a powdery form, or leave them coarse and natural.

Store the crushed tea leaves in a covered, cool place. Do not leave them in the open, or store them in a wet and damp place. You can use two techniques to store Moringa leaves for tea: a) you can put them in individual tea bags for quick use, or b) you can store them in a container together. Kept in a secured place, the tea could have a shelf life of more than 6 months.

To actually prepare Moringa tea, boil water in a kettle. Add 2 tsp of Moringa leaf powder into the kettle and let it come to a boil. Separate the powder/excess leaves from the water with a strainer and pour it into a teacup. Add lemon juice and/or sugar.

However, since most of the times, Moringa tea is used for weight loss purposes, perhaps it will be better if you substitute sugar with artificial sweetener or pure honey.

If you are using Moring teabags, dip the bags into hot water in a cup; mix lemon juice and/or honey to taste.

Another simpler way to make Moringa tea is simply to boil 1/4 cup of raw and cleaned Moringa leaves in 1 cup of water and strain it to drink.

The taste of Moringa tea might seem a little bitter for someone who is trying it for the first time, but adding honey and lemon juice will make it better.

ii. Moringa Smoothie

Moringa smoothie can be made with adding 1 or 1/2 teaspoon of Moringa leaf powder in any regular that you drink regularly. However, if you want to emphasize on this nutritious if not delicious powder, here's a smoothie recipe that would be perfect for you. You will need:

- 1/2 of a pineapple, fresh and ripe
- 3 tbsp of Moringa powder (the same powder that you used for tea)
- 2 pears, fresh
- 1.5 cup of coconut milk
- 1/8 cup of lemon juice, freshly squeezed

Chop up the pineapple and the pears into big chunks. Add all the ingredients together in a blender and mix until smooth. Pour into a glass and enjoy!

If you are new to the taste of Moringa or not completely comfortable with the taste, reduce the amount to 1 tsp. or 1/2 tsp. of the powder. Slowly increase the amount as you go on.

Here's another Moringa smoothie recipe that you will enjoy too. For this, you will need:

- 1 tbsp of Moringa leaf powder (the same powder)
- 1 whole banana, ripe

- 1 Date

- 2 tsp cacao powder

- 1 tbsp almond butter, melted at room temperature

- 1/2 cup of coconut water (not coconut milk, but water from a green coconut)

- 2 tbsp lemon juice, freshly squeezed

- A few ice cubes

Add all the ingredients to your blender and process until smooth. You can also add a little honey to the mixture. Add the ice cubes to the glass or into the blender, if it could take the pressure.

iii. Moringa Juice

If you are not a smoothie person, but prefer lighter and simpler juices, this is the perfect recipe for you. You will need:

- 1 carrot, large

- 1 tbsp of Moringa powder

- 1 grapefruit, squeezed

- 1 tbsp honey

Cut the cleaned carrot into small chunks and grind them in a mixer. Alternatively, you can grate them into shreds. Put the carrots into a juicer or a blender and blend until smooth. Add a little water if you need a little help in breaking them down.

Strain the blended carrot to separate the juice from the pulp. Add the Moringa powder and the grapefruit extract. Add honey to taste. You can also add a little mint to the juice for some extra flavor.

Basically, you can add a little Moringa powder to any other fruits and vegetables to make juice, such as ginger, celery, berries, spinach or cucumber.

iv. Moringa Chicken Salad

Moringa is above all, a health food and the best way to eat it is with some other healthy dish - a salad, for example. Next we have a chicken salad recipe where we could incorporate fresh Moringa leaves beautifully. You will require:

- 1.5 cup of Boneless chicken meat, cooked or boiled

- 1/2 cup of Moringa leaves, freshly picked

- 4 tbsp mayonnaise

- 1/4 cup onions, finely chopped

- 1/4 cup celery, finely chopped

- 1 tsp Cayenne Pepper

- 2 tbsp Worcestershire sauce

- Sea salt or Garlic salt

- Italian seasoning

Mix all the ingredients together. Add the salt and the seasoning according to your taste. You can also squeeze a little lemon juice on it before eating.

This mixture of chicken, mayonnaise and Moringa leaves can also be used as a filling for cold sandwiches served as snacks.

v. Moringa Coleslaw

Speaking of healthy food, here's another recipe for Moringa-based coleslaw that you can eat as a salad, or use as a dip with your fried snacks. You will need:

- 1/3 cup cabbage
- 1/4 cup carrots
- 1/4 cup onions
- 2 cloves of garlic
- 1/4 cup air-dried Moringa leaves
- 1/3 cup mayonnaise
- 1/2 tsp sea salt
- 2 tbsp vinegar

Shred the cabbage, carrots and the onions and mix together. Add to it the salt and mayonnaise. Using your hand, crumble the dried Moringa leaves and add to the dish. Top with the vinegar and mix well to serve.

vi. Moringa Soup

Moringa leaves or powder added to any soup increases its nutrition manifold. Here is a recipe of a simple vegetable soup that will help you get through a cold evening at home or during a fever. You will need the following ingredients:

- 1 cup vegetable broth, or 1 piece vegetable bullion
- 1/2 cup fresh Moringa leaves
- 6 tsp of soy sauce

- 1 celery stick, sliced

- 8 nos. button mushroom, fresh

- 2 carrots, small and sliced

- 1 onion, small and finely chopped

- 2 liters of water

Boil the water and add the vegetable stock/bullion. After the two ingredients mix together well, add the chopped onion and the sliced celery sticks and carrots. Add the mushrooms.

Cover the pan and cook in medium heat for around 20 minutes. Add the Moringa leaves and bring to a boil for 2 more minutes. Serve hot.

MORINGA BEAUTY PREPARATIONS

Moringa is not only good for your health, but also for your skin and hair, as we have learned in detail in the previous chapters. Here we have a few skin and hair care products that can be made using parts of the Moringa Oleifera plant that will help your skin glow and your hair shine.

vii. Moringa Oil Sleep Treatment

This is a massage oil that, if used at night before going to bed, will give you a good night's sleep and a peaceful rest. To make the oil at home, you will need:

- 2 ounce of Moringa seed oil
  (oil extracted from the seeds of the Moringa plant)

- 2 ounce of Rosehip oil

- 3 tbsp of Evening primrose oil

- 5 tsp of Castor oil

- 3 Vitamin-E capsule Extracts

All the above mentioned types of oil can be found in any store that sells Essential oil and other beauty products. Make sure that you buy oils that are raw and pure.

Put all the ingredients, one after another, in a small dropper bottle and use the stirrer to mix them well together. At night, before going to sleep, apply the oil to your face, neck, shoulders, and especially on your temples and forehead. Massage in with your hands.

This can also be used for aromatherapy during a full-fledged massage.

viii. Moringa Tea Facial Mask

Another great way to use Moringa is by applying a facial mask. This is the perfect way to nourish and moisturize your skin, especially if you are prone to acne and dryness. You will need:

- 4 Moringa tea bags, or 5 tsp of Moringa leaf powder

- 1 tsp baking powder

- 3 tsp rice flour

- Water

Add all the ingredients together (take out the Moringa tea powder if you are using tea bags). Mix them all in and add a little powder to make a thick paste. Gently, using your hands, apply this paste to your face and neck. Leave it on for 20-25 minutes, without moving your face muscles too much, i.e. laughing, talking, etc.

When the mask starts to dry, wash it off with lukewarm water. Apply moisturizer. Your face will be feeling fresh, clean and soft.

ix. Moringa Tea Hair Care Oil

Now, it is time to care for your hair using Moringa Tea. This miracle tea made from the leaves of the Moringa plant can help bring back the shine to your dull hair, making it stronger and healthier looking. This routine is best practiced when you are taking a shower, so keep the Moringa tea ready beforehand.

Brew 3 Moringa tea bags (alternatively, 4 tsp of Moringa leaf tea) in a kettle in 1 liter water for 10 minutes. Cool the tea in room temperature. When you are taking a shower, shampoo your hair to make it clean and wet.

Rinse your hair and your scalp with the cooled Moringa tea, taking slow and deliberate moves. Use your fingers, dipped in the Moringa tea, to gently massage your scalp - just as you would apply oil to your hair. Do this for a few minutes until all the tea is gone.

Wash your hair with running water for a few minutes, and then apply your regular conditioner. After drying, your hair will look shinier and bouncier, and feel stronger from within.

x. Moringa Oil Toner for Acne-prone Skin

Those who have suffered from acne all their life know exactly how painful and uncomfortable it is, and also how difficult to control. Using Moringa oil as toner, you can keep your skin clean, hydrated and bacteria-free, causing fewer breakouts. You will need:

- 4 tsp Moringa oil

- 2 tbsp Coconut Oil

- 1.5 cup of Witch Hazel Oil

Mix all the ingredients together in a plastic container, using a stirrer. Clean your face with your regular cleanser, and apply the toner to your face with the help of a cotton ball. Apply moisturizer.

If you have oily skin, reduce or omit the coconut oil. You can also include any other Essential oil that suits your skin. This toner will help you fight breakout as well as prevent wrinkles and premature aging.

OTHER MORINGA PREPARATIONS

Apart from cooking and beauty products, Moringa can also be used in making some other helpful objects to use around the house.

xi. Moringa Soap

Soaps made from Moringa leaves have anti-bacterial properties and can be used to wash your hands or your body, or to clean the house. It is easy to make and can be achieved in the kitchen with no troubles at all.

To make Moringa soap, you have to collect green, freshly picked Moringa leaves, and blend them in a mixer. The mixture has to be very smooth, so it may take a while to turn all the leaves into a pulp. You can also add a little water so that all the leaves are gone and turns into a smooth mash.

If the paste becomes too thick, add a little water to it. Using your hands, mix the leaf pulp and the water, and take out any excess leaf portion or stick that may still be in the mixture.

Now, strain the Moringa paste to extract the juice from it. You can use a very fine sieve to do the job, or a soft piece of cloth tied over a container. Make sure you get all the juice out so that you are left with a thick and dry pulp.

Add coconut oil to the mixture. You can use almost the same - or half - amount of Moringa juice that you have. Stir well, but only in one direction. Add a little perfume to the mixture something that is natural and has a strong scent, such as citrus.

Soak caustic soda in water overnight, and add to the mixture. The color would probably change at this point into light green; the juice will thicken too.

The final stage would be to pour the mixture into molds. You can use baking trays to do the job, and later cut of the soap bars in different sizes. Or, you could pour the soap mixture into bread pans, and cut out actual soap shaped bars later. Set aside until the soap mixture thickens.

When the mixture thickens enough, cut out the soaps in little bars with a knife. Or, you can have fun with your cookie cutters and cut off playful shapes to be used as soap in the toilet.

xii. Moringa Powder

Moringa leaves are the most versatile part of the plant, and can be used in cooking and creating a multitude of dishes. They are easy to make, easy to store as well as very very to use.

Collect some fresh Moringa leaves from a plant. Clean them in cool water so that they have no dirt or waste attached to them.

The next step would be to blanch the leaves. For those who are new to this, blanching is a process where you immerse any fruit or vegetable in extremely hot, boiling water to make it lose its flavor, color and taste to some extent. To blanch the Moringa leaves, hold them in boiling water not more than 5 seconds.

Place the leaves on a tray, and keep them in a shady but airy place to dry. Do not dry them directly under the sun, as that would reduce some of the main nutrition of the leaves. Turn over the leaves a few times to ensure proper air-drying.

When the leaves have completely dried, use your hands to crumble them into small particles. You can also rub them over a fine strainer until you have the desired uniformity.

This is a multi-purpose powder than can be used in almost any cooking as a condiment or spice. You can sprinkle this at the end of cooking every meal, regardless of whether it is vegetable, poultry, cattle or fish. This powder can also be used in baking pizza, quiches, brownies or muffins.

You can also use this powder to brew tea, or add it to any drink, i.e. a smoothie or a juice. Only a spoonful of Moringa leaf powder would be enough to ensure the nutritional needs of any adult for a whole day.

Check Out Joy's other book:

Essential Oils Guide for Beginners: The #1 Natural Resource for Weight Loss, Anti-Aging, Natural Cures, Healthy Lifestyles

See the book here:

http://www.amazon.com/Essential-Oils-Beginners-Anti-Aging-Aromatherapy-ebook/dp/B00UIEMIRG

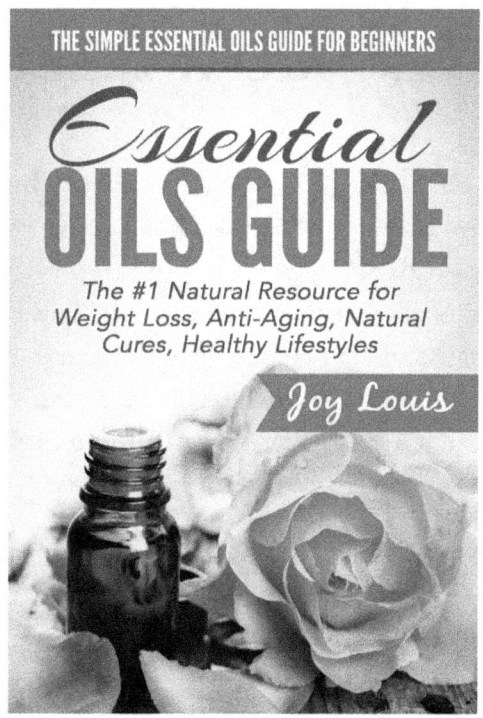

DO YOU LIKE FREE BOOKS? Find out how we can you send you FREE BOOKS BELOW!

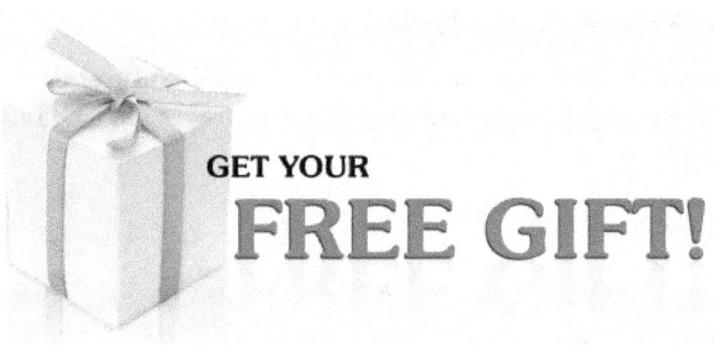

GET YOUR

FREE GIFT!

WAIT! – DO YOU LIKE FREE BOOKS?

My **FREE Gift** to You!! As a way to say **Thank You** for downloading my book, I'd like to offer you more **FREE BOOKS!** Each time we release a NEW book, we offer it first to a small number of people as a test - drive. Because of your commitment here in downloading my book, I'd love for you to be a part of this group. You can join easily here → **http://goo.gl/4lB2sj**

Do You Enjoy **FREE BOOKS**? Do you like books that are Life Changing, Inspirational, Motivational and Informative? We **LOVE** sharing **FREE BOOKS** with people like you. It's easy to join just by clicking here → **http://goo.gl/4lB2sj**

CONCLUSION

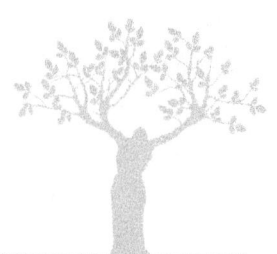

Thank you again for downloading this book!

I hope this book was able to help you to get excited about essential oils.

The next step is to look for more books on essential oils and natural living.

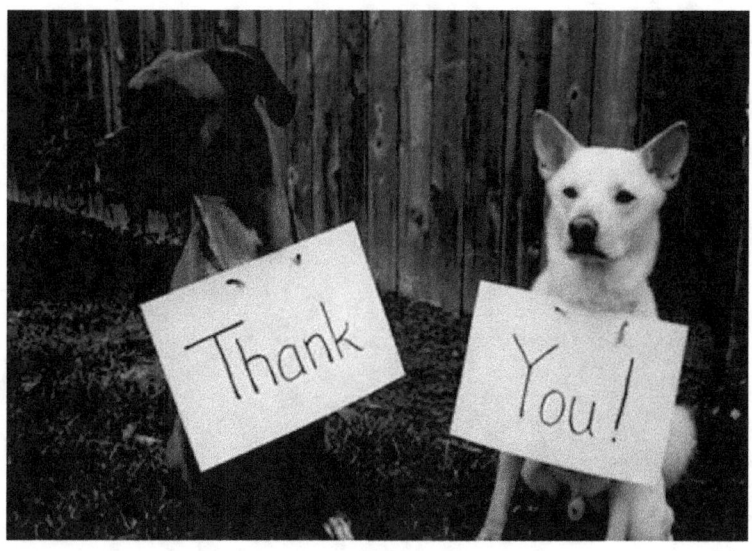

Finally, if you enjoyed this book, then I'd like to ask you for a favor, would you be kind enough to leave a review for this book on Amazon? It'd be greatly appreciated!

Help us better serve you by sending questions or comments to joylouisbooks@gmail.com - Thank you!